Dr. Oumou DIAKITE

Medical and nutritional therapy for kidney diseases

Dr. Oumou DIAKITE

Medical and nutritional therapy for kidney diseases

SciencíaScripts

Imprint

Cover image: www.ingimage.com

This book is a translation from the original published under ISBN 978-620-6-72593-0.

Publisher:
Sciencia Scripts
is a trademark of
Dodo Books Indian Ocean Ltd. and OmniScriptum S.R.L publishing group

120 High Road, East Finchley, London, N2 9ED, United Kingdom
Str. Armeneasca 28/1, office 1, Chisinau MD-2012, Republic of Moldova, Europe
Managing Directors: Ieva Konstantinova, Victoria Ursu
info@omniscriptum.com

Printed at: see last page
ISBN: 978-620-8-41024-7

Tebla of contents

Medical and nutritional therapy for kidney diseases

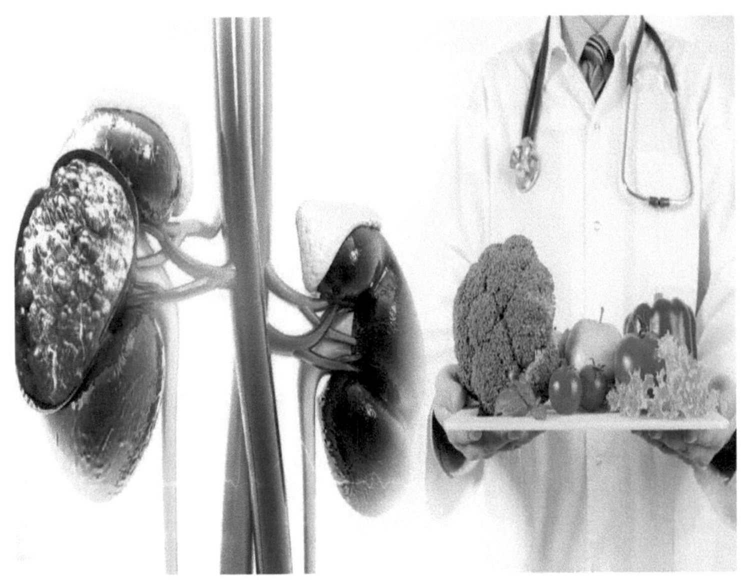

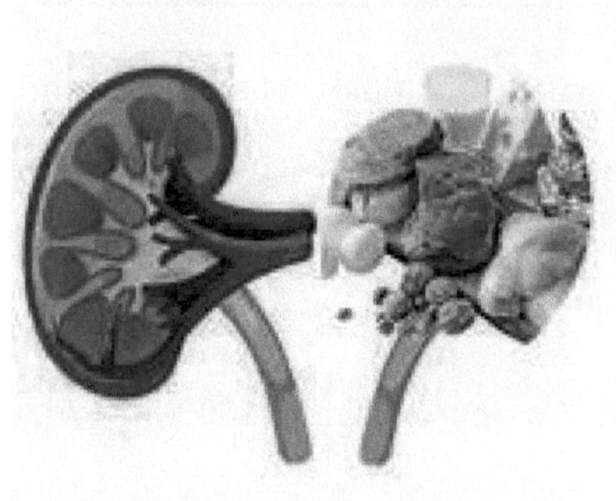

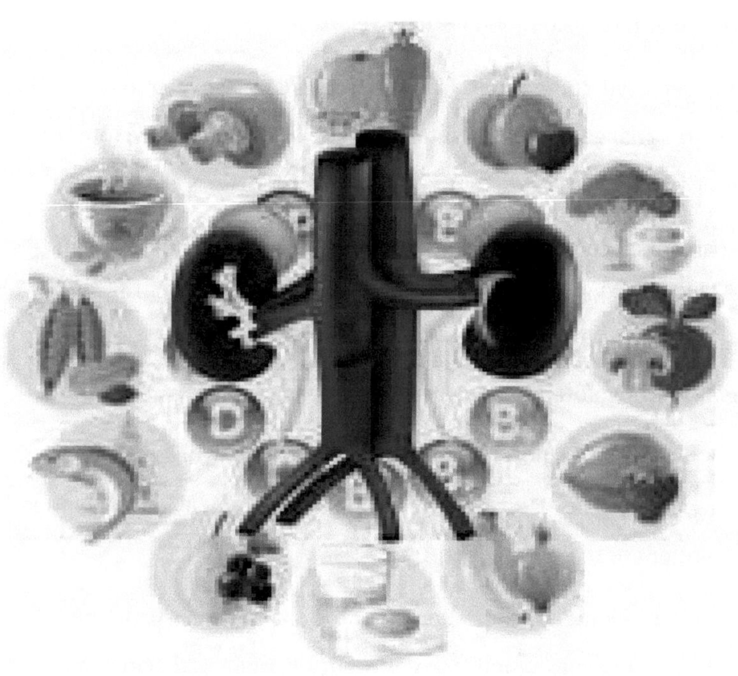

I- Kidney physiology and function:

Maintaining the balance of fluids, electrolytes and organic solutes is the kidney's main function. This function is ensured by blood filtration. The kidney receives 20% of cardiac output. An adult has 5 liters of blood.

The blood filtered is approximately 1600 liters/day and 180 liters of ultrafilter liquid.

There are two (2) kidneys, located dorsally in abdomen on the last two (2) ribs on either side of the spine. The right kidney is slightly lower than the left, to accommodate the liver.

Some secreted components are reabsorbed by active transport. This leads to a change in the ultrafilter fluid (1.5 liters of urine excrete for an average of 1 day).

The architecture of each kidney is marvellous, and is composed of one (1) million nephrons making up the glomerulus, connected to series of tubules including the proximal convoluted tubule, the loop of Henle, the distal convoluted tubule and the collecting tubule.

Each nephron functions independently, and is involved in the final production urine. Destruction a nephron segment leads general impairment of the entire nephron.

The renal glomerulus is the nephron's proximal structure. The glomerulus receives blood from afferent arteriole and sends it to the efferent arteriole. Thanks to its relatively high pressure, this network enables formation of primitive urine, also known as ultrafiltrate. Together with Bowman's capsule, it forms Malpighi's corpuscle.

Vasopressin, known as antidiuretic hormone (ADH), secreted by the magnocellular nuclei of the posterior pituitary, regulates water . An excess of relative body water, indicated by low osmolarity, causes all vasopressin secretions to cease rapidly.

Vasopressin is an oligopeptide formed by the union of 9 amino acids, including cysteine, tyrosine, glutamine, proline, an amine group, phenylalanine, arginine, asparagine and a carboxyl group.

It has a certain influence on the cardiovascular and central nervous systems, among others.

Calcium-phosphorus homeostasis is maintained by complex interactions parathyroid hormone (PTH); calcitonin; active vitamin D.

Calcitonin is the hormone whose function is to reduce calcium levels in the blood. It is secreted in response hypercalcemia and has at least two effects: suppression of renal tubular reabsorption of calcium. In other words, calcitonin increases calcium excretion in the urine.

The effector organs of this homeostasis maintenance are the intestine, kidneys and the liver.

bones.

The kidney's role includes the production of the active form of vitamin D 1,25- dihydroxycholecalciferol (1,25[OH] 2D3), as well as the elimination of calcium and phosphorus.

Calcium absorbed from the intestine by active vitamin D. The latter is necessary for bone remodeling and maintenance.

Active vitamin D also abrogates the production of PTH, which is responsible for mobilizing calcium from the bones.

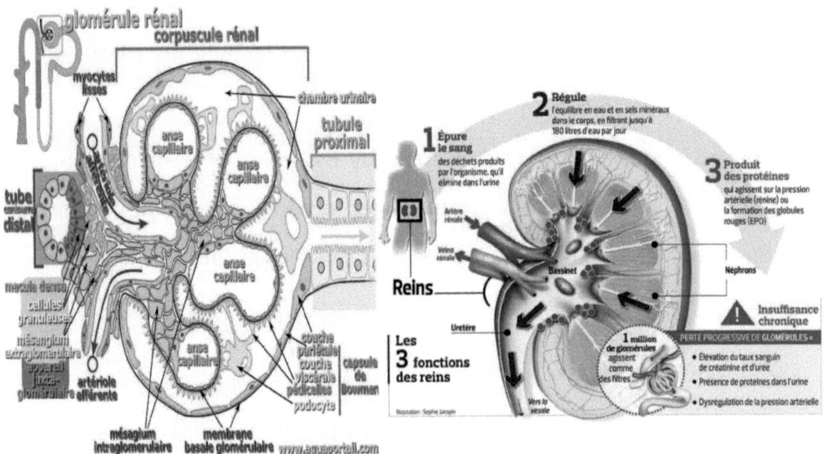
glomérule rénal
corpuscule rénal
myocytes lisses
chambre urinaire
tubule proximal
anse capillaire
anse capillaire
anse capillaire
anse capillaire
tube
distal
macula densa
cellules granuleuses
mésangium extraglomerulaire
appareil juxta-glomérulaire
artériole efférente
couche pariétale
couche viscérale
pédicelles
podocyte
capsule de Bowman
mésagium intraglomerulaire
membrane basale glomérulaire
www.aquaportail.com
1 Épure le sang
des déchets produits par l'organisme, qu'il élimine dans l'urine
2 Régule
l'équilibre en eau et en sels minéraux dans le corps, en filtrant jusqu'à 180 litres d'eau par jour
3 Produit des protéines
qui agissent sur la pression artérielle (rénine) ou la formation des globules rouges (EPO)
Artère rénale
Veine rénale
Bassinet
Néphrons
Reins
Uretère
Les 3 fonctions des reins
Vers la vessie
Insuffisance chronique
PERTE PROGRESSIVE DE GLOMÉRULES =
1 million de glomérules agissent comme des filtres
• Élevation du taux sanguin de créatinine et d'urée
• Présence de protéines dans l'urine
• Dysrégulation de la pression artérielle

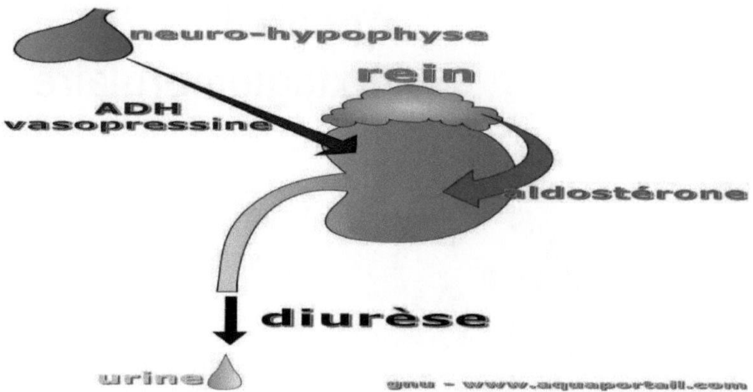

1-The juxtaglomerular apparatus :

The juxtaglomerular apparatus is a functional association of cells within the kidney. It is juxtaposed by the glomerulus of the kidney particles. It enables renal regulation electrolyte balance, as well as systematic programming blood pressure regulation.

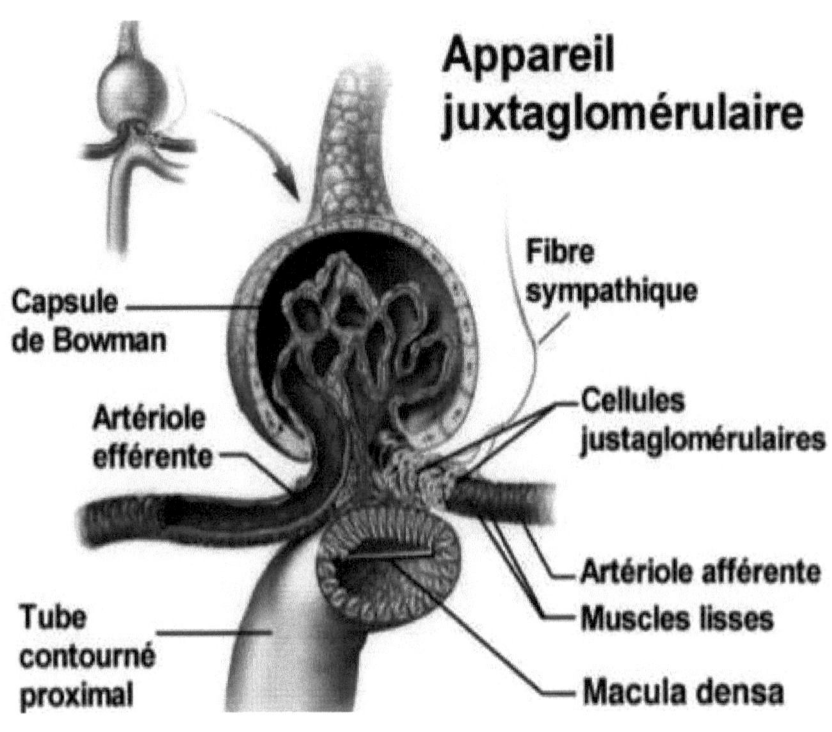
Appareil
juxtaglomérulaire
Fibre
sympathique
Capsule
de Bowman
Artériole
efférente
Cellules
justaglomérulaires
Artériole afférente
Muscles lisses
Tube
contourné
proximal
Macula densa

Nutritional consultation and

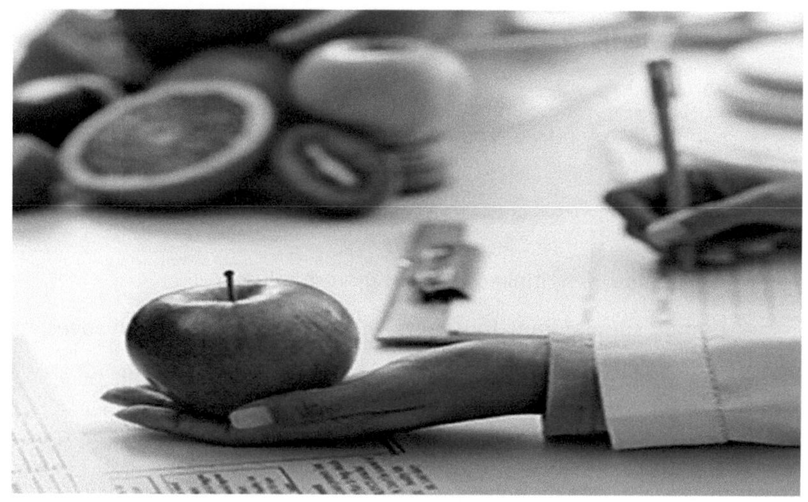

Nutritional and dietetic consultation:

I- Story:

It must include the patient's current state of health and diagnosis.

Essential information can be :

- ✓ date of first diagnosis
- ✓ Previous education according to diagnosis
- ✓ Recent diagnostic procedures speak of NPO (Nothing By mouth) in the fasting patient.
- ✓ Dentition, chewing or swallowing difficulties, chronic gastrointestinal symptoms (diarrhea, constipation, nausea, vomiting).
- ✓ Family history relevant to the disease, the onset of the pathology and patient's age.
- ✓ Surgical history
- ✓ Variations in multiple drugs and their duration.
- ✓ Dietary supplements (nutrients, infusions, tree roots and leaves, essential nutrients) and their uses, which can be chronic or as-needed.
- ✓ Symptoms of changes smell and taste caused by the use of medicines
- ✓ The patient's personal information (age, gender, cultural and ethnic identification, income, lifestyle, occupation, and ability to perform daily activities).

II- Physical examination in nutrition :

nutritional status through procedures of ingestion, digestion, absorption, transport and metabolism. Identifying the signs and symptoms associated with nutrient deficiency and malnutrition must be our goal.

In 2010, the international committee developed etiology-based approach to the diagnosis of adult malnutrition in the clinical setting.

The latter may be encountered in acute or chronic pathologies or injuries, and may be linked to a starvation etiology.

The 6 keys unlocking the door to diagnosing malnutrition in in adults are :

1. Weight loss
2. Insufficient energy intake
3. Loss of subcutaneous body fat
4. Loss of muscle mass
5. Fluid accumulation that can mask weight loss
6. Decreased functional status (unable carry normal activities) of the day).

Nutritional evaluation

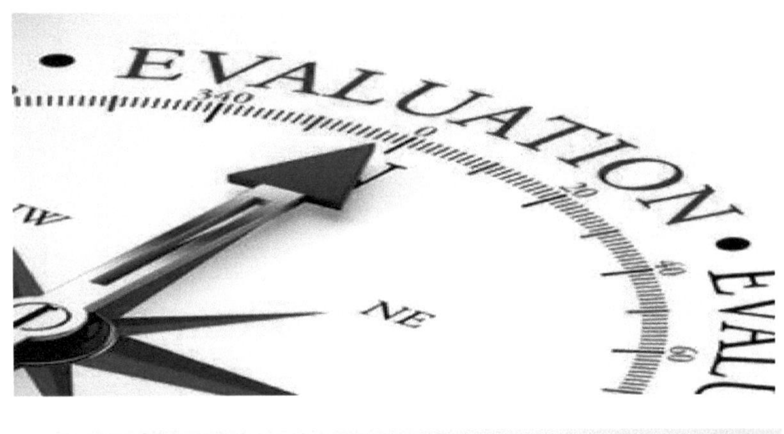

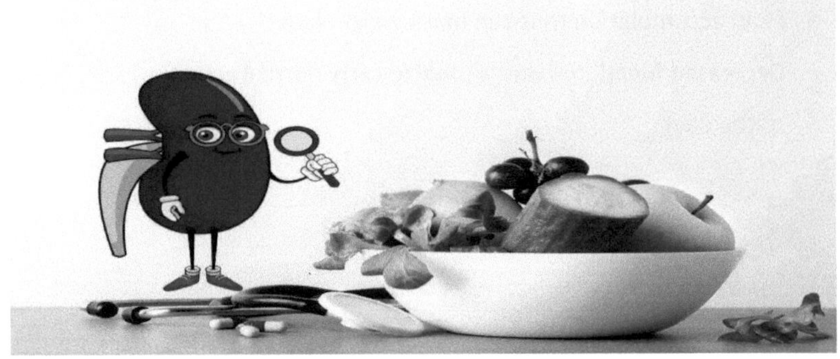

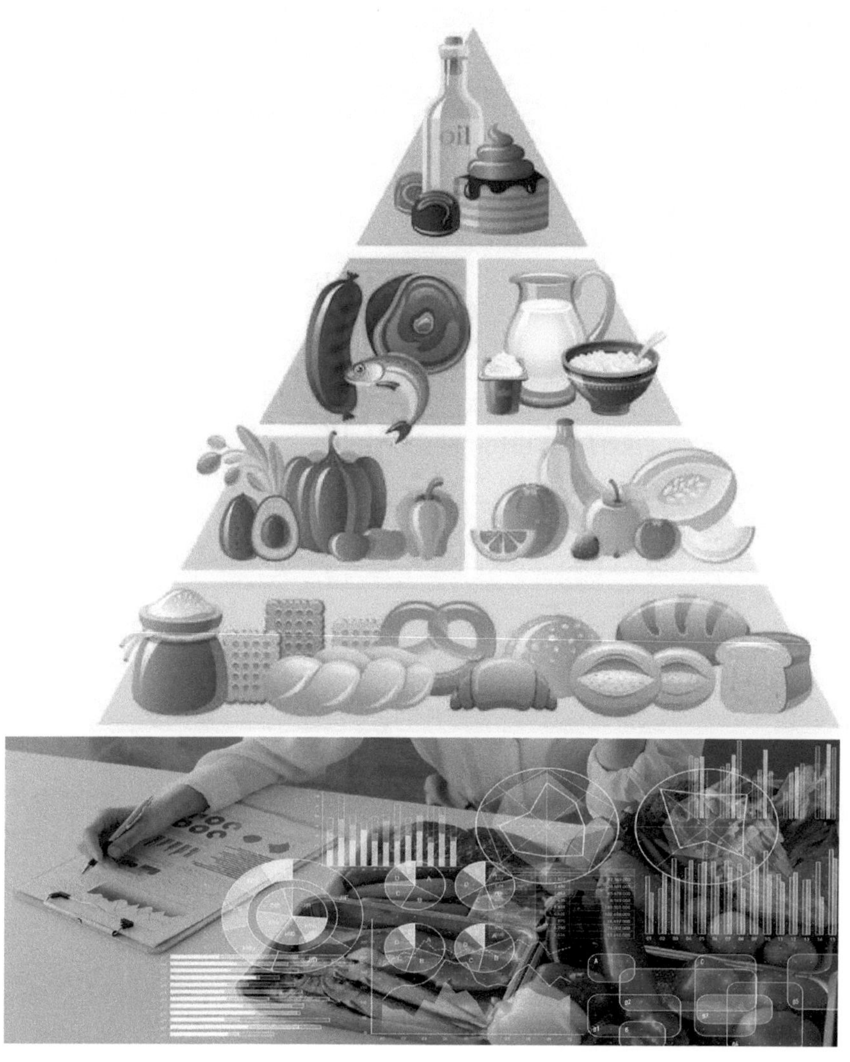

Nutritional evaluation :

Patient name :_______________Date of entry :

Gender :___________________Date of birth :   Name of Nutritionist :

Size :   Weight :   Ideal weight :   Recent weight/weight gain :

Ethnicity : ___ Religion :

Diagnosis (physical and mental) :__________________________

Snack scheme : Food from external sources :

Need self-help devices : ______ Consumption:

Previous plan :

Where food is taken: Dining room : Tray in room :

Appetite : Diet prescription : ________Date:

Food or vitamin supplement :

Diet history: Ability to chew and swallow :

Skin (decubitus or subject to skin breakdown) :

Vision and hearing :   physical limitations

Kidney disease proper

I- The urinary tract includes :

- The kidneys, paired bean-shaped organs that urine
- The, the channels that urine from the kidneys to the bladder
- The bladder, a hollow organ contains urine until miction
- The urethra, a channel connected to the bladder that allows urine to flow out of the body. The difference between men and women is shown by the presence of the prostate, the penis in men and the vagina and vulva in women.

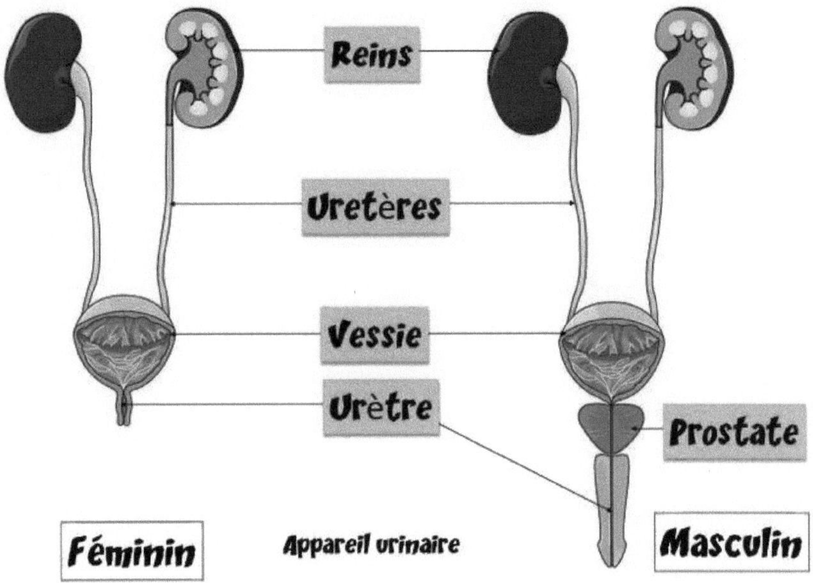

I- **Renal pathologies :**

We can classify kidney diseases according to their degree of severity:

- Kidney stones
- Acute kidney injury
- Chronic kidney disease
- End-stage renal disease

The development of nutritional care is linked to the treatment of pathologies

underlying factors.

A- **Kidney stones:**

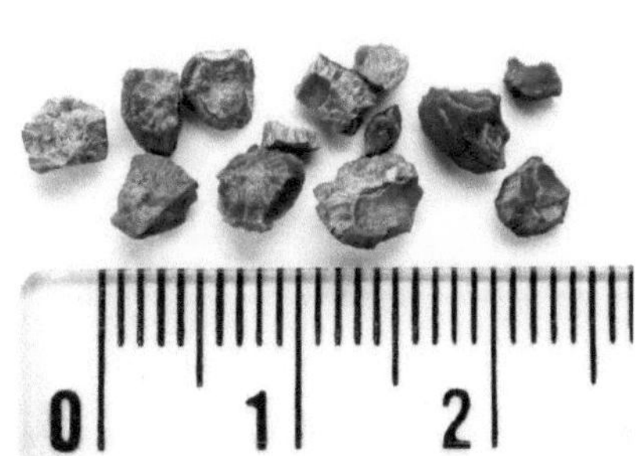

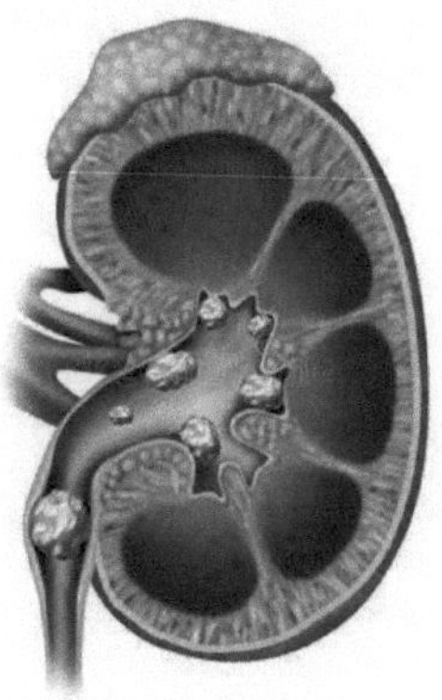

A kidney stone or urinary lithiasis is a solid concretion formed in the kidneys. It is composed of mineral salts and proteins and can measure up to 2 cm. Kidney stones are often referred to as "kidney stones". " [1]

A kidney stone is a small, hard crystal that forms in the kidney. It can be invisible to the naked eye or over 2.5 cm in diameter. Sometimes kidney stones remain in the kidneys and cause no symptoms. Sometimes, they leave the kidneys and move into the urinary tract. [2]

According to the author, a kidney stone is defined by the presence of a solid formation, mobile or not, of calcium, uric acid and cystine origin, with a variable size of 2.5 cm or more, blocking the normal flow of urine.

- **Types of kidney stones:**

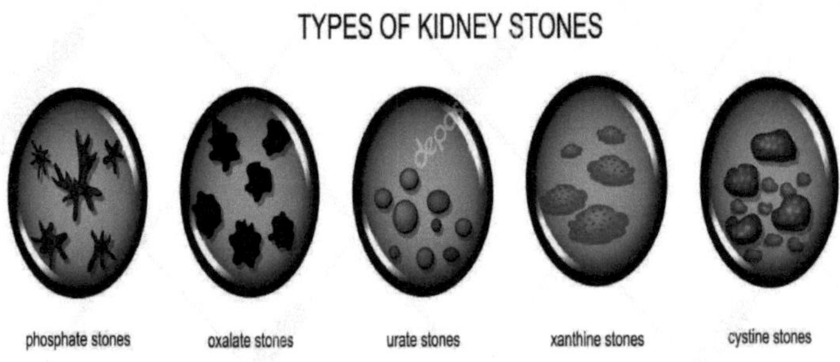

B- Acute kidney injury :

Acute kidney injury is a rapid decline in renal function occurring within days or weeks, leading to an accumulation of nitrogen products in the blood (formerly called uremia) with or without a reduction in the amount of urine produced. [3]

It is often the result of inadequate renal perfusion due medical pathology or surgery, or severe trauma, but sometimes it is triggered by a rapidly progressing intrinsic nephropathy.

Preliminary symptoms nausea, anorexia and vomiting. Convulsions and coma may follow, reflecting the consequences of lack of treatment. Fluid and electrolyte imbalances and disturbances of the acid-base balance rapidly develop.

Diagnosis is made with biological tests of renal function, including creatinine levels. Urinary indices, urine sediment examinationimaging and other tests (sometimes including renal biopsy) are necessary to determine the cause.

Treatment focuses the underlying etiologies with management of fluid and electrolyte balance, and sometimes dialysis.

C- Chronic kidney disease :

Chronic kidney disease (CKD) refers to the more or less severe impairment of kidney function, whatever the cause. The kidneys lose their ability to filter the body's blood properly, in a lasting and irreversible way.

Chronic kidney disease is a silent disease for a long time, with progressive evolution and no possibility of cure. [4]

Diagnosis based on ultrasound, biopsy, blood and urine tests (essential for confirming deterioration in renal function).

Levels of biochemical substances in the blood generally become abnormal when loss of kidney function reaches a certain level in chronic kidney disease. Urea and creatinine levels are increased, and the blood becomes moderately acidic. Potassium levels rise, and calcium and calcitriol levels fall. Phosphate and parathyroid hormone levels increase with anemia.

D-End-stage renal disease :

End-stage renal disease is the final stage of chronic renal failure. The kidneys no longer function well enough to meet the needs of daily life.

The kidneys of people with end-stage renal disease function at less than 10% of their normal capacity, which can mean they barely function or not at all. [5]

E- Kidney cancer:

Symptoms of kidney cancer may include :

- ✓ Hematuria: Presence of blood in the urine, which can lead to the appearance of a blood clot.

  pink or reddish color.
- ✓ Pain in the flank or lower back: Persistent or stabbing pain on the side of the affected kidney.
- ✓ Palpable mass: You may feel a lump or mass in the kidney area.
- ✓ Unexplained fatigue: Persistent fatigue for no apparent reason.
- ✓ Unexplained weight Weight loss without any change in diet or physical activity.
- ✓ swelling of the ankles or legs.

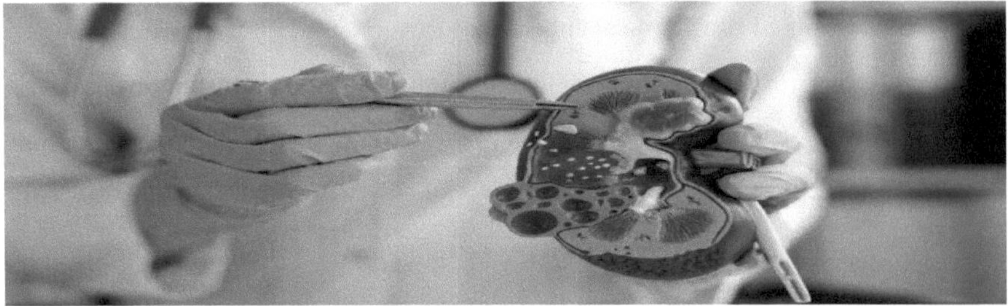

Malignant tumors (cancer):

- ✓ Clear-cell carcinoma is the most common type.

- ✓ It mainly affects men between the of 50 and 70. When it develops at a young age, a genetic mutation (VHL gene mutation) is sought.

- ✓ Papillary carcinoma, frequently diagnosed in patients with renal failure. High-grade forms may be genetic in origin (FH mutation).

Chromophobe carcinoma: better prognosis, but often large in size

Some tumors can be benign (20% of kidney tumors):

- ✓ Oncocytoma
- ✓ Angiomyolipoma.

What are the stages of kidney cancer?

In stage T1, the kidney tumor measures a maximum of 7 cm in diameter. It is located in the kidney.

In stage T2, the tumor measures over 7 cm in diameter, but remains localized in the kidney. It has not spread to lymph nodes or other tissues.

At stage T3, the tumor now affects the major blood vessels (renal vein and inferior vena cava). It may also affect neighboring tissues or lymph nodes.

In stage T4, the tumor has spread outside the kidney. It affects the adrenal gland, distant lymph nodes or other organs.

Tumors are also classified according to their grade. This classification makes it possible to assess the speed of spread of cancer cells. [6]

causes of malignant tumours are: smoking; obesity; high blood pressure; family history of kidney cancer; radiotherapy treatment. Women treated with radiotherapy for genital cancer have a slightly higher risk; certain genetic mutations, notably in the VHL, FH, MET and FLCN genes; prolonged dialysis treatment.
Von Hippel-Lindau disease. People with this hereditary disease are at greater risk of developing kidney cancer.

Diagnosis: is based on a CT or MRI scan of the abdomen. This determines the size of the kidney tumour. It also identifies the stage of the kidney cancer (metastasized, regional or local).

Once the diagnosis has been confirmed, the patient is treated by a urological surgeon. In most cases of renal cell carcinoma, surgery is performed.

This is used to remove the tumour and confirm the diagnosis. If this is not possible, a biopsy is performed. The tumor or tumor sample is then analyzed in a laboratory. This determines the type and grade of cancer.

Imaging tests are carried out in cases of metastasized kidney cancer: chest CT scan, bone scan, brain CT or MRI. These tests look for metastases in the lungs, bones and brain.

Treatment of kidney cancer depends on the patient's stage and state of health. Surgery is the first-line treatment most kidney cancers, whatever their stage. It may involve partial or total nephrectomy (removal of part or all of the affected kidney). Lymph nodes or the adrenal gland may also be removed. Minimally invasive approaches are preferred (laparoscopy and robot-assisted surgery

The oncologist may recommend radiotherapy if the disease has metastasized. Radiotherapy is mainly used to relieve the symptoms of kidney cancer, notably pain. Targeted therapies block the development of cancer cells. It is administered if surgery is not possible, or as an adjuvant treatment (after surgery). In this case, it reduces the risk of recurrence. Immunotherapy aims to stimulate the immune system to destroy cancer cells on its own. Chemotherapy is rarely used for kidney cancer.

It is important to comply **with medical follow-up** after kidney cancer treatment. This ensures rapid treatment in the event of recurrence. Follow-up usually involves clinical and imaging examinations, and blood tests. Follow-up lasts several years.

This medical article has been reviewed and validated by a doctor specializing in oncology at an ELSAN facility, one of France's leading private hospitalization groups. It is intended for information purposes only and in no way replaces the opinion of your doctor, who is the only person authorized to make a diagnosis.

To establish a precise medical diagnosis for your personal case, or to find out more about your pathology, we remind you that it is essential to contact and consult a doctor.

Therapeutic nutrition and kidneys

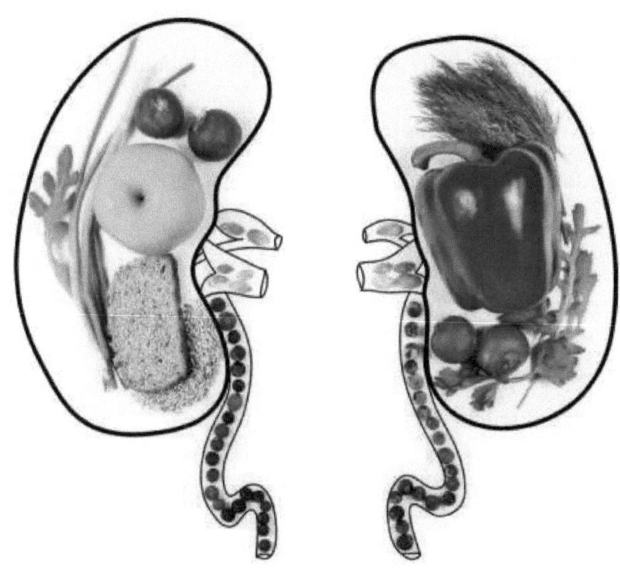

Our diet plays a very important role in the health of our kidneys, especially in the treatment of chronic renal failure and other kidney diseases.

The creation of a daily nutritional plan is of paramount importance. This plan depends on the factors involved, and will ensure a fulfilling and healthy life for patients kidney disease. Renal function must be assessed during appointments, and the diet adapted according to the degree of severity of the renal pathology.

Therefore, the need for dietary changes will depend on blood tests.

A diet in question will meet nutritional needs; preserve kidneys by decreasing their function; control the accumulation of food waste (urea in your blood); reduce symptoms (fatiguenausea, itching and a bad taste in the mouth).

Nutrient monitoring to minimize symptoms of kidney disease and stabilize blood pressure with excellent health:

PROTEINS: form, repair and maintain the body's tissues. They fight infection and help heal wounds. As your body breaks down protein foods, urea is formed. Failure to eliminate urea causes the kidneys to double up, leading to fatigue, nausea, headaches and a bad taste in the mouth.

Protein consumption is therefore an excellent remedy for kidney treatment. Protein is found in milk, eggs, legumes, nuts, fish, poultry and lean meat.

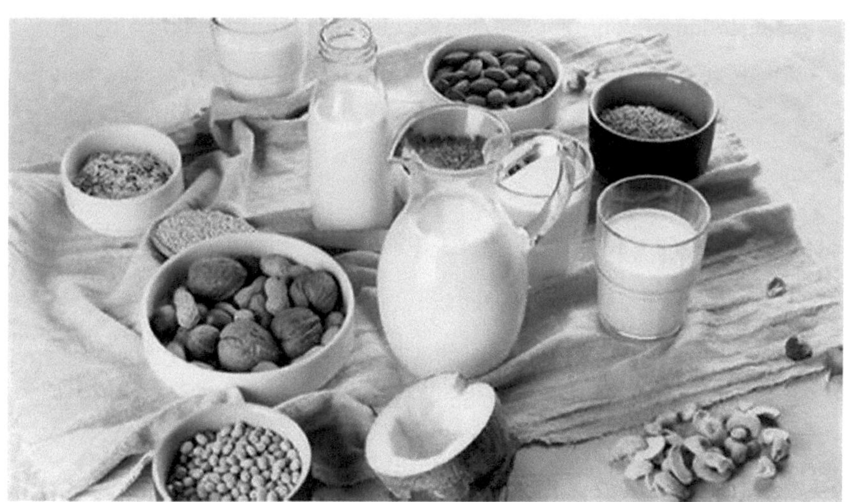

SODIUM

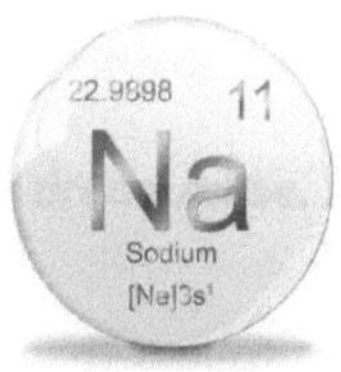

What you eat has a direct effect on your kidneys. Your diet is therefore a very important part of your treatment plan for chronic kidney disease. Your dietary needs are unique and depend on many factors, including your current kidney function, your other health problems (diabetes, hypertension, etc.), your medications, your weight and your general state of health.

Creating a daily nutritional plan that takes all these factors into account will help you feel good about yourself, and constant modification of your diet will find excellent modification in the health of your kidneys. Blood tests should be taken at all times to ensure that the regimen is progressing smoothly. A diet suitable for the kidneys can:

- meet your nutritional needs;
- preserve your kidneys by reducing their workload;
- help control the accumulation of food waste, such as urea, in your blood;
- minimize the symptoms, such as the fatigue, the nausea, itching and a bad taste in the mouth.

As your kidney function deteriorates, your body is less able to remove excess sodium from your blood. This sodium can raise your blood pressure and cause swelling in your ankles and legs. People chronic renal failure should generally limit their salt intake to less than 2000 mg per day (one teaspoon of salt contains 2300 mg of sodium). The best way to do this is to replace processed foods with homemade ones, so you can control the amount of salt you take in. Processed foods such as deli meats, snacks, fast foods, canned vegetables, cheese, pickles and condiments all have added salt. Even bread and other baked goods often contain salt. So be sure to read food labels. When cooking at home, using pepper, onions, garlic, lime, lemon or vinegar to season your food.

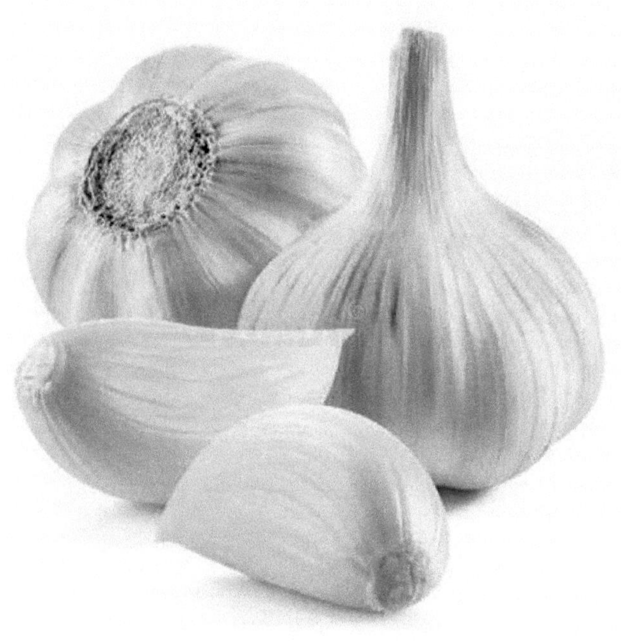

PHOSPHORUS (PHOSPHATE)

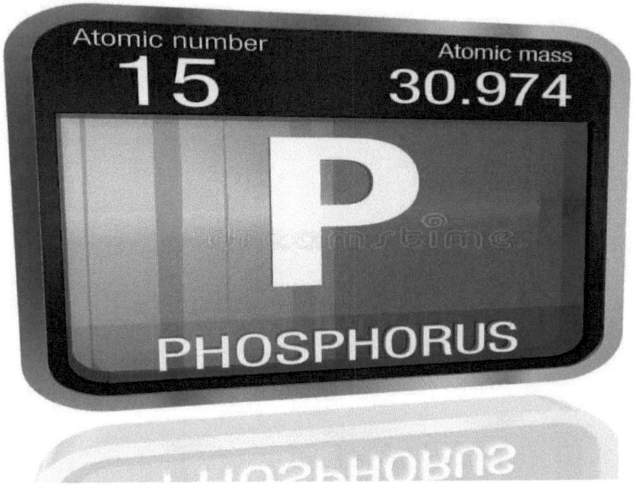

Phosphorus is a mineral that keeps your bones strong and healthy. Too much phosphorus, however, can cause itching or joint pain. When your kidneys begin to fail, the phosphate level in your blood increases. At this stage, you may need to limit foods containing phosphorus, especially those to which phosphates are added to extend shelf life or improve taste. Your dietician will ensure that phosphates are limited and that patients receive the other nutrients they need to stay healthy. Your doctor may also prescribe phosphate binders (these drugs, often calcium-based, bind to the phosphate in the food you eat) also known as phosphate agglutination . These drugs bind to the phosphorus in your intestine and the phosphorus passes into your stools.

A diagnosis of chronic kidney disease doesn't necessarily mean you have to follow a boring or bland diet. The daily nutrition plan you develop with your dietitian can include all kinds of fresh, delicious foods. Don't hesitate to talk to your dietitian and take advantage of Cuisine et santé rénale to add variety to your meals. Bon appétit!

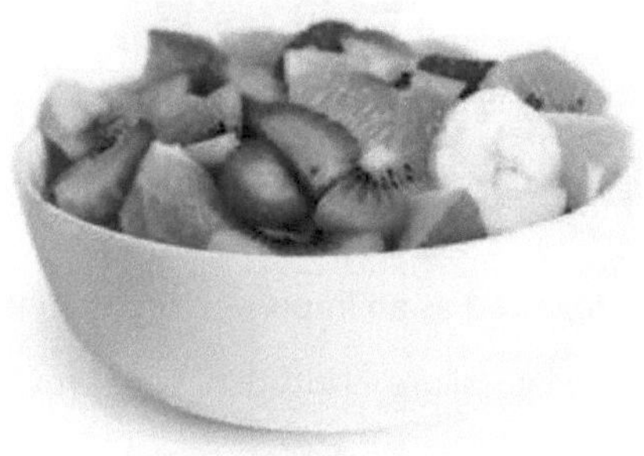

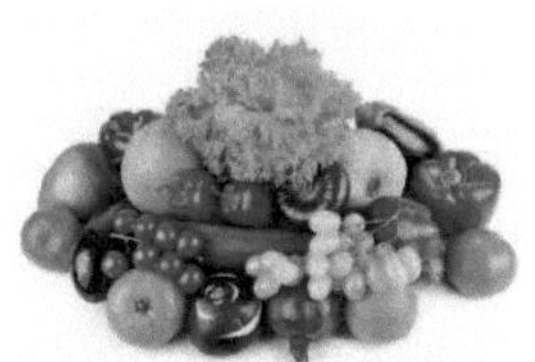

Sensitive studies have been carried out detailing relevant relationships between a healthy diet and healthy kidneys.

Fruits and vegetables

Studies show that a plant-based diet is beneficial to renal health. Patients with chronic renal failure who modify their diet to reduce its acid load (by increasing fruit and vegetable consumption) see metabolic acidosis improve and the progression of their renal disease delayed. Thus, increasing fruit and vegetable consumption improves metabolic acidosis and kidney damage to the same extent as oral sodium bicarbonate supplementation.

7 aliments qui nettoient naturellement les reins

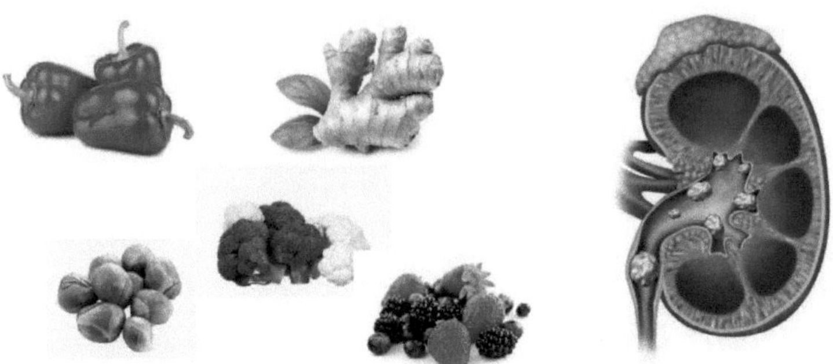

Oxidative stress is increasingly recognized as an important factor in the onset and progression chronic renal failure. Nutrition can provide antioxidants, particularly through fruit and vegetables, to combat the damage caused by free radicals.

Among the antioxidants found in plants is sulforaphane in cabbage: broccoli, cauliflower, kale, Brussels sprouts... Cabbages reduce damage to the organs affected by complications of type 2 diabetes, such as the liver and kidneys. However, some cabbages such as Brussels sprouts are also rich in potassium, excretion of which is impaired in advanced chronic renal failure; patients are often advised to limit their intake to avoid potentially fatal hyperkalemia.

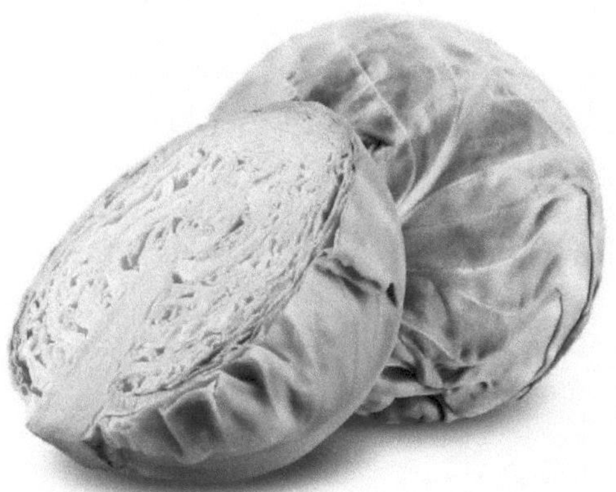

In addition to vitamin C, polyphenols among the natural antioxidants found in plants. They are found in large quantities in red berries, black grapes, strawberries, blueberries, raspberries, etc. Among fruits, berries (wild blueberries, blackberries, bilberries, raspberries, strawberries) and pomegranates have the highest antioxidant activity.

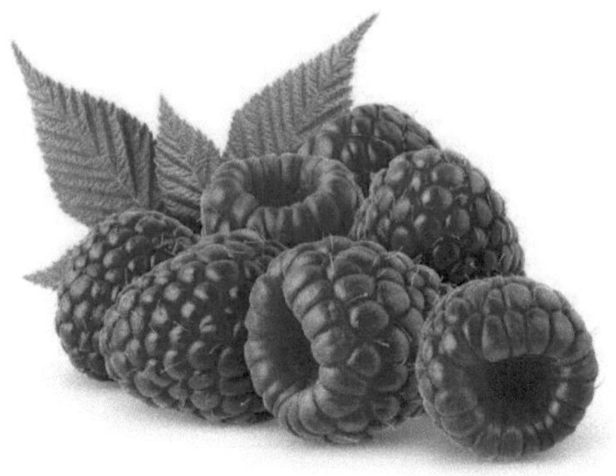

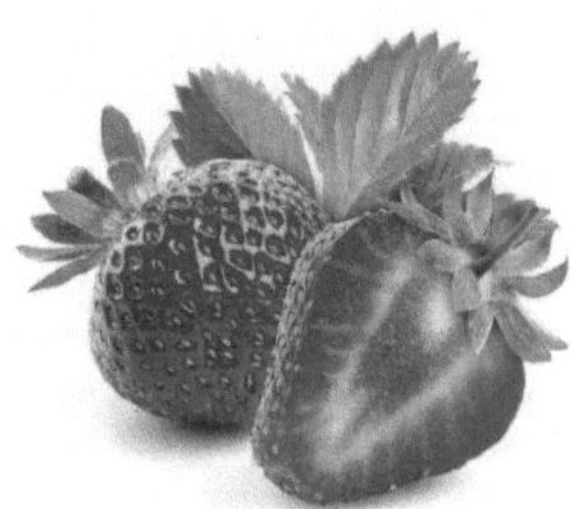

Olive oil is also rich in antioxidants.

Against urinary tract infections: cranberry

Cranberries contain proanthocyanidins, molecules that inhibit the adhesion of Escherichia coli bacteria to the urothelial cells lining the bladder. A Cochrane review confirms that cranberry-containing products help prevent urinary tract infections. According to its authors, cranberry juice and cranberry-based supplements reduce the risk recurrent urinary tract infections by more than a quarter women, by more than half in children, and by around 53% in people prone to urinary tract infections following medical procedures.

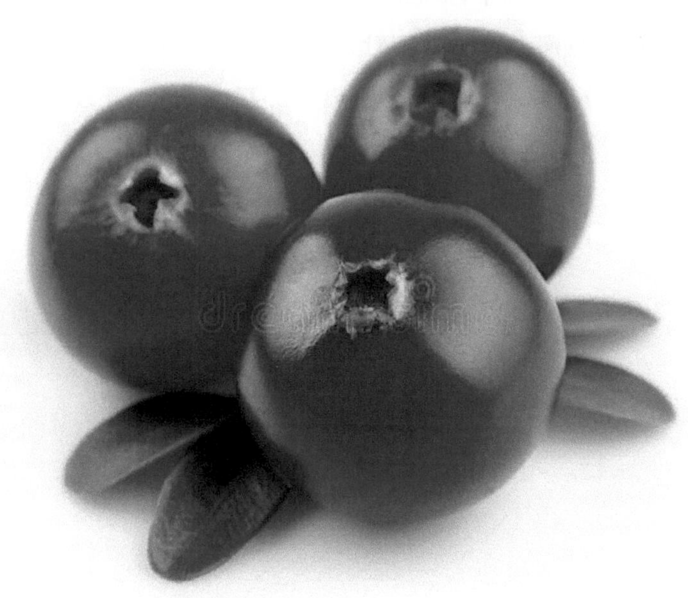

Moderate protein intake

In the case of renal failure, it is generally advisable to limit protein intake, as proteins are converted into urea, which can accumulate in the blood if the body has difficulty eliminating it. In a study of 1,594 patients suffering from kidney disease, researchers observed that the lower the initial protein intake, the slower the disease progressed. However, you shouldn't reduce your protein intake too much either, as the authors consider it dangerous to go below 0.6 g/kg per day.

Little salt

A kidney-healthy diet also avoids excesses of sodium (salt), potassium and phosphorus, as blood levels of phosphorus and potassium can rise in kidney failure. A low-salt diet limits the complications of kidney failure. In short, a typical Western diet, rich in salt, animal proteins and low in fruit and vegetables, should be avoided.

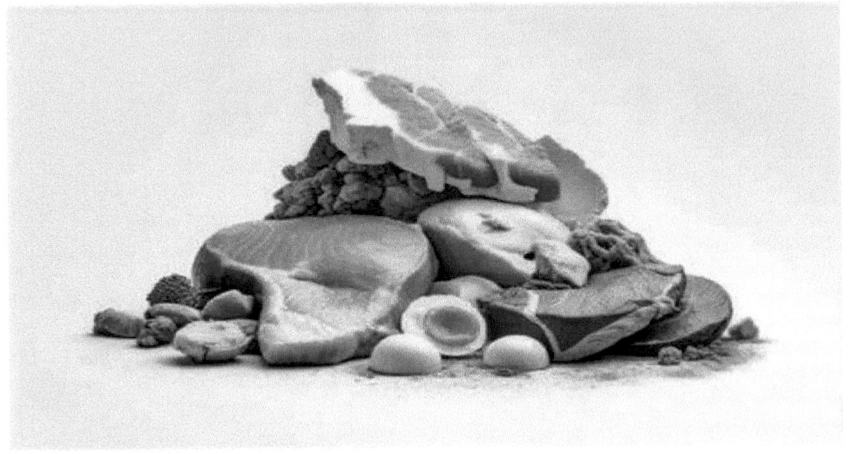

Montpellier University Hospital has published a brochure with dietary advice to protect the kidneys. The nephrology department advises patients not to exceed 6 g of salt per day (or 2.4 g of sodium). For phosphorus, the Anses has set the nutritional reference at 550 mg per day for adults, and 3.5 g for potassium.

Should I choose foods low in potassium?

Traditionally, diets for kidney disease were low in potassium. But, in 2022, researchers at New York University claim that "This recommendation was based on outdated research and often erroneous assumptions that do not reflect current data." Indeed, studies conducted over the past few decades show that patients kidney failure derive no benefit from restricting plant foods. "In general, there is no correlation between dietary potassium and serum potassium," say the researchers, "and we believe this is due to the effects of fiber on colonic potassium absorption, the alkalinizing effect of fruits and vegetables on metabolic acidosis, and the bioavailability of dietary potassium in plant foods." Ultimately, for them, dietary recommendations for renal health should be devoid of restrictions on dietary potassium contained in plant foods (10).

While potassium should not be in excess, it should not be in short supply , as it limits blood pressure and is alkalinizing, thus preventing kidney stones. In fact, kidney stones are the result of the crystallization of mineral salts and acids present in excessive concentrations in the urine. In Potassium mode d'emploi, Dr. Philippe Veroli explains: "Increasing dietary potassium intake reduces urinary calcium excretion and improves the calcium balance. This is how a high potassium intake reduces the risk of calcium kidney stones." Dietary acid load is the main risk factor for kidney stones (11). An alkalinizing diet, with a negative PRAL index, is therefore more favorable to renal health.

Discover below a video presenting the Reinbow app, created by Sandra Gressard, dietician-nutritionist and author of Bye Bye kidney stones.

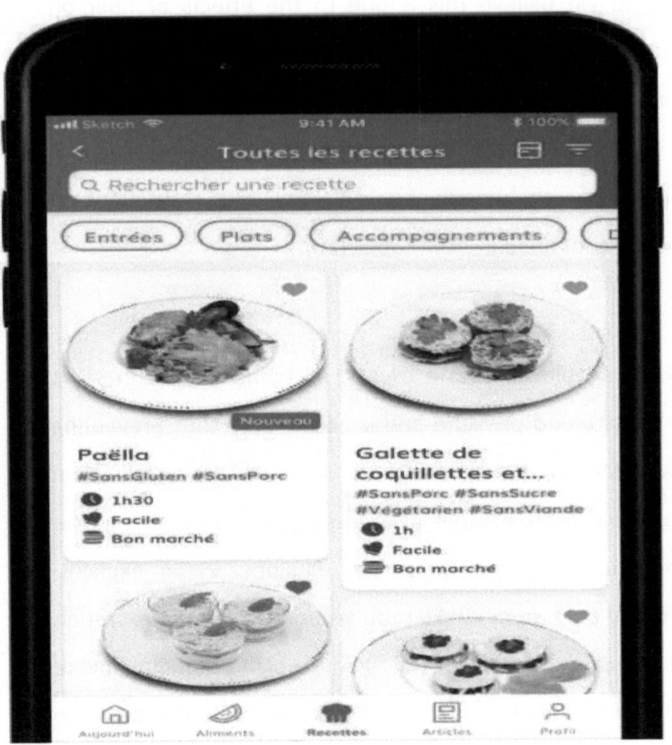

Aromatic plants, garlic and spices for seasoning dishes

To enhance the taste of dishes, use spices and herbs, which are generally antioxidant foods. Garlic is also a good option. In one study, garlic extracts protected the liver and kidneys from the deleterious effects of smoking.

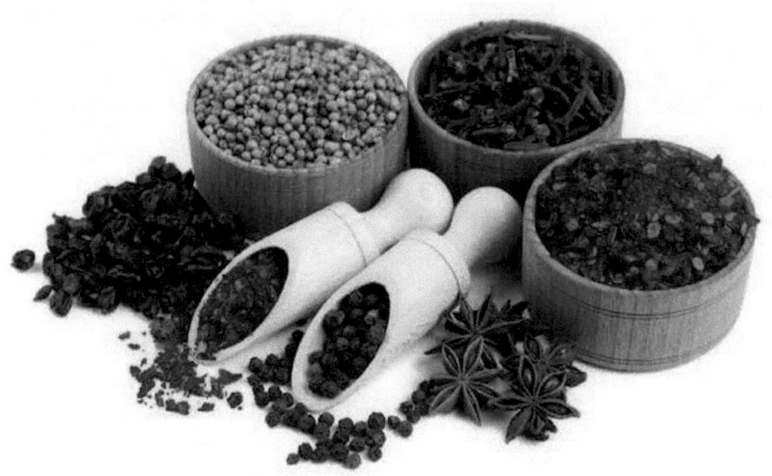

Among spices, ginger in particular appears to be protective of the kidneys. In an analysis published in 2022, Iranian researchers found that it reduced serum creatinine levels and diabetic kidney damage in animals (13). The authors conclude that "Ginger may improve glycemic indices, lipid profile, some inflammatory markers, oxidative stress and pathological lesions in diabetic kidney disease."

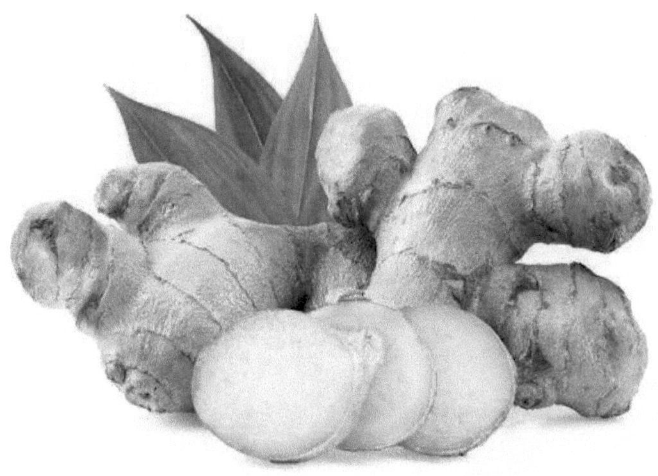

Water

Every day, the body needs around 1.5 L of water. This amount of water may vary in summer or according to your physical condition: "to avoid dehydration, you need to increase your water intake in the event of hot weather, intense physical activity (sport) or diarrhoea," explains the Montpellier University Hospital.

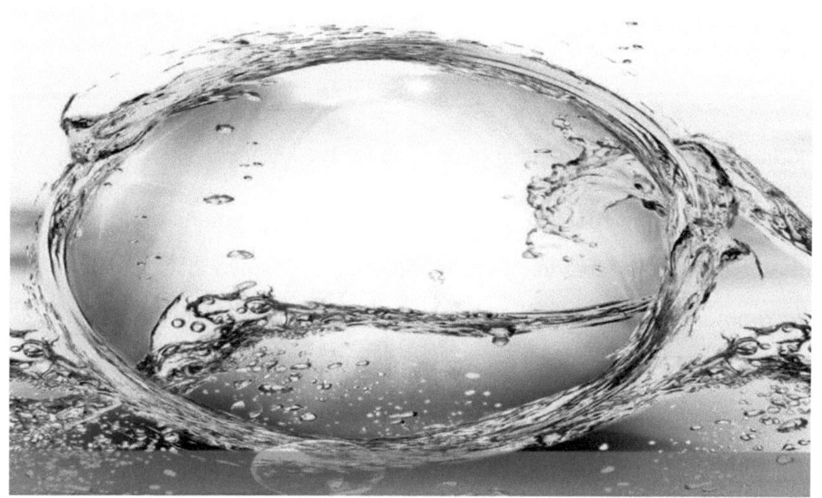

The most alkaline waters are those with the highest bicarbonate content, and are most often sparkling waters. If you drink sparkling water, sure it's not too high in salt, and choose a water with less than 50 mg of sodium per liter, such as Salvetat® or San Pellegrino®.

Is tea or coffee bad for the kidneys?
Tea and coffee provide antioxidants. However, drinking too much coffee is not recommended. A recent study carried out by the Universities of Toronto (Canada) and Padua (Italy) highlighted the kidney risks associated with three or more cups of coffee a day, in people who have difficulty metabolizing caffeine.

As Dr. Tamara Hew-Butler, a specialist in water balance, explains, "while alcohol has diuretic properties - ethanol acts directly on the kidneys to increase the amount of urine produced - caffeinated beverages, like tea and coffee, don't increase fluid loss through urine beyond what they contain."

Kidney detox: what's the best herbal tea for the kidneys?

Like the liver and the skin, the kidney is one of the emunctory organs that eliminate waste. In phytotherapy, linden sapwood is generally recommended for draining the kidneys. You can combine it with heather flowers, which are diuretic, urinary antiseptic and anti-inflammatory, and goldenrod flowering tops. Bearberry is also recommended against urinary tract infections. [7]

The Hospital

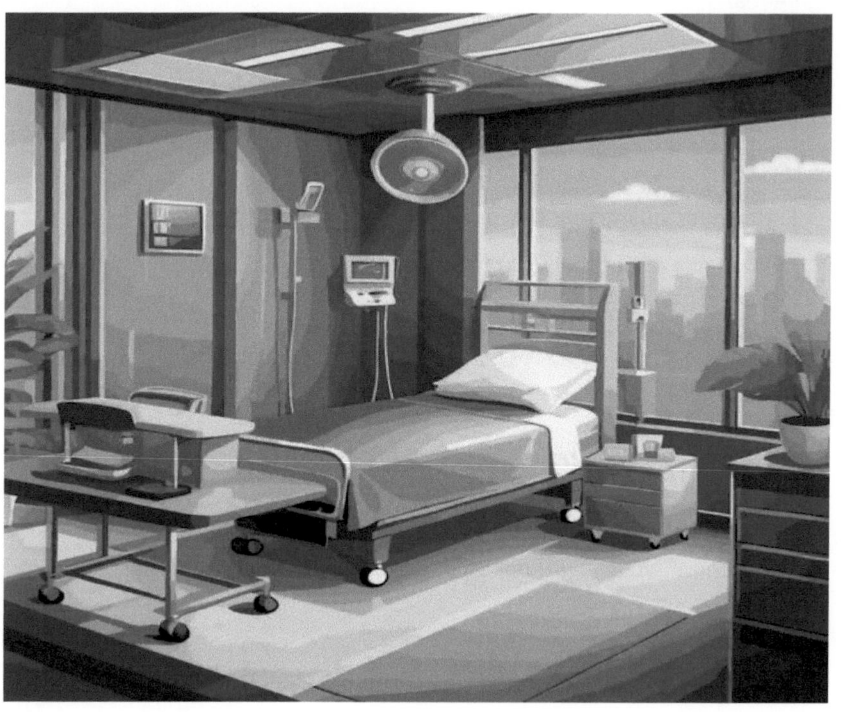

During treatment, some days may be better than others for your appetite. Large meals may seem too heavy or unappetizing. This can happen if your appetite decreases (you feel less like eating than usual) or if you feel full more quickly (you feel satisfied soon after you start eating).

Here are a few suggestions to help you get the most out of your meals.

Eat smaller quantities, but more frequently. For example, eat 6 to 8 meals a day rather than 3 large meals.

Eat every few hours. Don't wait until you're hungry.

Serve smaller portions on dessert plates instead of regular plates.

Drink hot chocolate, high-calorie fruit juices and nectars.

Avoid low-calorie beverages such as water, coffee, tea and diet drinks. To prepare your own milkshakes and milk-based drinks, see the "Recipes" section.

Make sure you always have your favourite snacks at home, on the move and at work.

Eat your favorite foods at any time of day. For example, have breakfast (such as toast or eggs) for lunch or dinner.

To make them more appetizing, incorporate different colors and textures.

in your meals.
To make your meals even more enjoyable, enjoy them with your loved ones in a place that's just right for you.

peaceful and relaxing.

Prepare foods that smell good, such as pastries or fresh bread.

Tips for increasing protein in your diet

To function properly, your body needs a balance between calories and protein. Your doctor or dietician may ask you temporarily increase your protein intake. If you've recently had surgery or have scars, eating more protein will help you heal. Below are some suggestions help you increase your protein intake.

Favor protein-rich foods such chicken, fish, pork, beef, lamb, eggs, milk, cheese, beans, nuts or vegetable butters, and soy products.

Drink condensed milk and use it in recipes instead of milk or water, for example in instant cakes, cocoa, omelettes and pancake batter. To prepare condensed milk, mix 1 envelope (about 1 cup) of fat-free milk powder with 1 liter of whole milk in a blender. Store in the fridge.

Use condensed milk or ready-to-drink food supplements (e.g. Ensure®) in your hot or cold cereals.

Add cheese and diced cooked meat to your omelettes or quiches.

Add unflavored protein powder to cream soups, mashed potatoes, smoothies and stews.

Spread your rusks with cheese or oilseed butter (peanut, cashew, almond , etc.).

Coat apples, bananas or celery with nut butter. Try apple

slices covered with cheese and honey.

Add nut butter to smoothies or shakes. Nibble on walnuts, pumpkin seeds or sunflower seeds.

Add nuts and seeds to breads, muffins, pancakes, cookies and waffles.

Try hummus on pita bread. Use hummus as a spread on sandwiches or add a spoonful to salad.

Add cooked meats to soups, stews and salads.

Sprinkle your cereals, casseroles and yoghurts with wheat germ, peanuts, chia seeds or ground flax seeds.

Choose Greek-style yoghurt rather than ordinary yoghurt.

Eat desserts made with eggs, such as four- quarters, puddings, custards and cheesecakes.

Put more eggs or egg whites in your custards, puddings, quiches, pancake batter, French toast, scrambled eggs or omelettes.

Add grated cheese to sauces, vegetables and soups. You can also use it on baked or mashed potatoes, casseroles and salads.
Add fresh cheese or ricotta to stews and casseroles.
pasta or eggs.

Put melted cheese on burgers and breaded cutlets. Sprinkle your salads

with chickpeas, kidney beans, tofu and hard-boiled eggs,
nuts, seeds and cooked meat or fish.

Use pasteurized bone for soups and stews.

Tips for increasing calorie intake in your diet

Here are a few suggestions to help you eat more calories. They may seem to contradict you already know about healthy eating. But during treatment and throughout your recovery, the most important thing is get enough calories and protein.

Avoid foods and beverages labelled "low-fat", "fat-free" or "diet". For example, choose whole milk rather than skimmed milk.

Snack on dried fruit, nuts or seeds. Add them to cereals, ice creams or salads.

Drink fruit nectars or smoothies.

Add butter, clarified butter or oils to , rice and pasta. Do the same with cooked vegetables, sandwiches, toast and cereals.

Add spreadable cheese or oleaginous butter to toast, slices of bread or vegetables.

Spread your cookies with creamy cheese, jam or peanut butter.

Spread jelly or honey on bread or cookies.

Mix jam with fruit salads and use as a topping on ice cream or cakes.

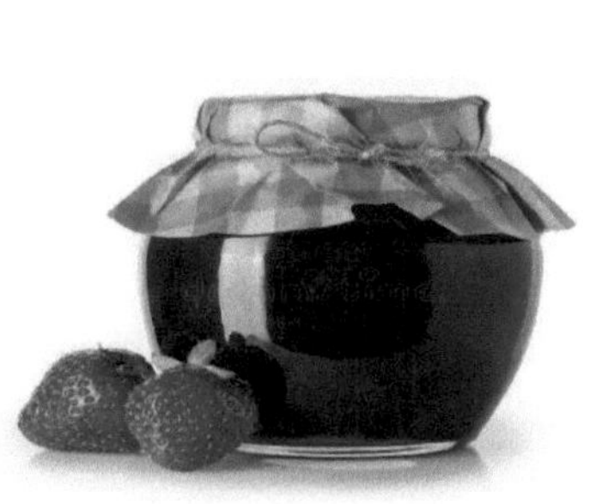

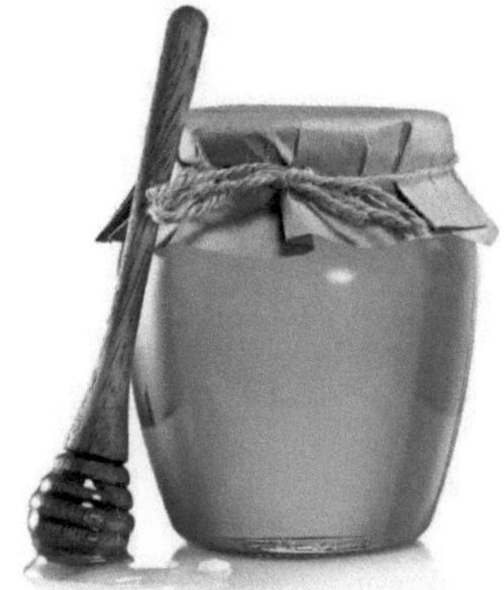

Dip tortilla chips in guacamole or tangy cream sauce.

Use high-calorie dressings on salads, baked potatoes and vegetables (green beans and asparagus, for example).

Add sour sauce, coconut milk or heavy or semi-heavy cream to mashed , cakes and cookies. You can also add it to pancake , sauces, soups and simmered dishes.

Top baked potatoes with cheese or sour cream.
Add whipped cream to cakes, waffles, French toast, fruit, puddings and hot chocolate.

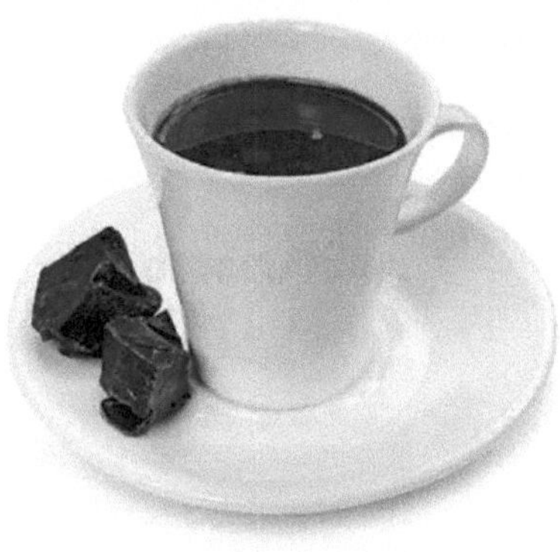

Before eating, garnish your vegetables and pasta with cream sauces. or a drizzle olive oil.

Add mayonnaise, creamy vinaigrette or aioli to your dishes.

salads, sandwiches and vegetables.

Put muesli in yoghurts, and on ice cream or fruit. Also use in cookie, muffin and bread doughs.

Top your ice cream or cupcakes with sweetened condensed milk. For more calories and flavor, combine condensed milk with peanut butter.

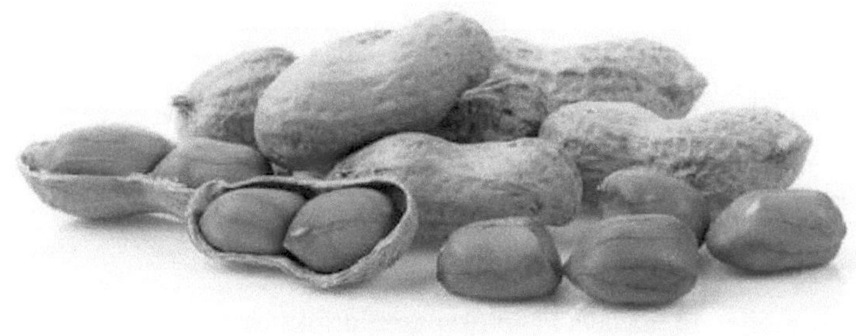

Add croutons to your salads. Accompany

your meals with fillings or garnishes.

Drink homemade milkshakes. Try the smoothie recipe in the "Recipes" section. You can also drink high-calorie, high-protein beverages (e.g. Carnation® Breakfast Essentials or Ensure®). You'll find a list of commercially available food supplements in the next section.

Add avocado to smoothies, soups, salads, omelettes and other dishes.

as a spread on toast.

Add mayonnaise or sour cream to your salads.

tuna or eggs, for example) or your sandwiches.

Back to top Food

supplements

If you don't know how to make your own smoothies, there are plenty of nutritional supplements on the . They come in the form of , high-calorie drinks to which vitamins and minerals have been added. They also come in powder form for mixing with other foods or dissolving in drinks. Most are also lactose-free, which means you can take them even if you're lactose-intolerant (have difficulty digesting dairy products).

Once opened, always keep prepared drinks refrigerated. Do the same with powders after mixing them with liquids.

Bland, tasteless drinks

These drinks are useful for anyone who likes moderately sweet tastes. They can be used as a base for lightly sweetened milkshakes. These drinks are :

- Lactose-free
- Gluten-free
- Kascher

Dietary supplement (manufacturer) Nutritional value

Osmolite® 1 Cal (Abbott)

Per 240 ml serving :
250 calories

10.5 grams

Isosource® HN

protein (Nestlé)

Per 240 ml serving :

300 calories

13.5 grams of

unscented Glytrol®

protein (Nestlé) Per

240 ml serving :

250 calories

11.3 grams of protein

Sweetened flavoured

drinks

These drinks are available in several flavors: vanilla, chocolate, strawberry and other flavors, depending on the brand. These drinks are :

- Lactose-free
- Gluten-free
- Kascher [8]

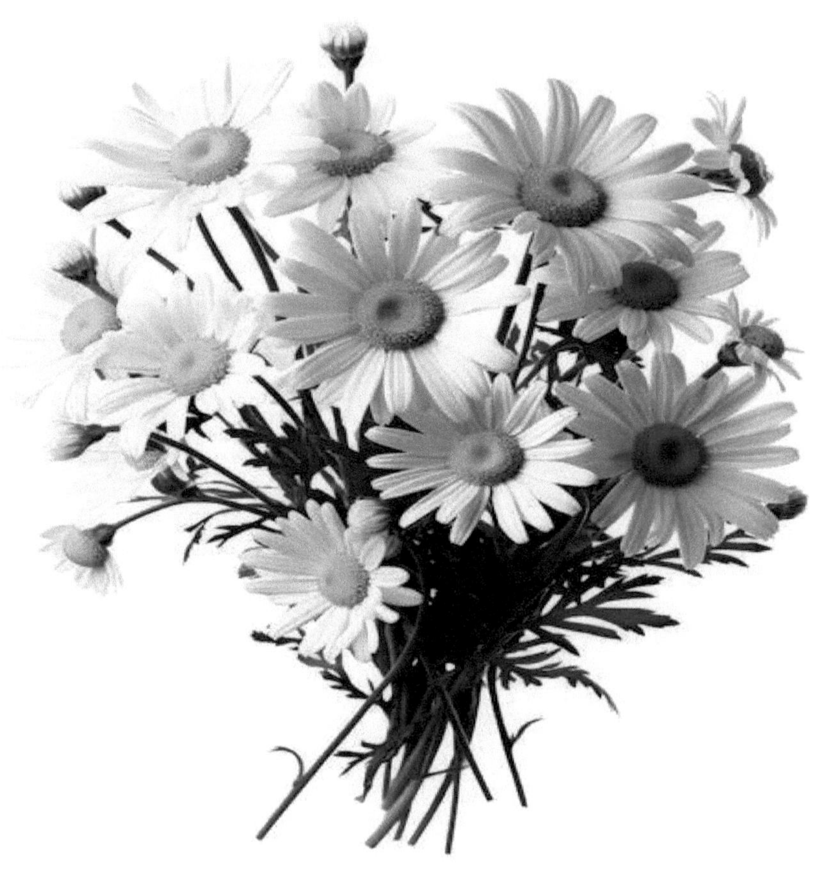

IN ALLAH WE BELIEVE

1- https://www.elsan.care/fr/pathologie-et-traitement/maladies-urinary/kidney calculations [1]
2- https://www.msdmanuals.com/en/home/the-facts-in-breath-disturb- r%C3%A9nals-and-urinary-vessels/calculations-in-urinary-vessels/calculations-in-urinary-vessels-calculations-r%C3%A9nals#:~:text=Un%20calcul%20r%C3%A9nal%20est%20u n%20p etit%20cristal%20dur,reins%20et%20se%20d%C3%A9placent%20 dans%2 0les%20voies%20urinaires. [2]
3- https://www.msdmanuals.com/fr/professional/troubles-g%C3%A9nito- urinary/l%C3%A9sion-r%C3%A9nale-acute%C3%AB/l%C3%A9sion- r%C3%A9nale-acute%C3%AB-insufficiency-r%C3%A9nale-acute%C3%AB[3]
4- https://www.ameli.fr/assure/sante/themes/maladie-renale-chronique[4]
5- https://genialsante.com/maladie-renale-en-phase-terminale-causes-symptoms-and-prevention/ [5]
6- https://www.elsan.care/fr/pathologie-et-traitement/cancers/cancer-du-kidney-definition-symptoms-treatments [6]
7- https://www.lanutrition.fr/quels-sont-les-aliments-bons-pour-les- kidneys[7]
8- https://www.mskcc.org/fr/cancer-care/patient-education/eating-well-during-your-treatment#section-3 [8]

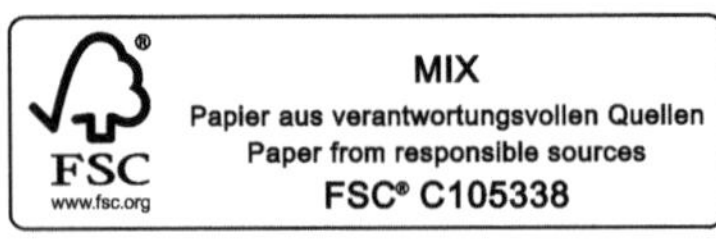

Printed by Books on Demand GmbH, Norderstedt / Germany